STARTING YOUR MEDICAL PRACTICE

For Beginners

Dee Whitelocke

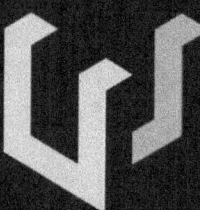

PRO INITIATIVE BILLING SVCS.

Table of Contents

INTRODUCTION

The decision to open a medical office, believe it or not, is the easy part. Aside from realizing your business plan's potential, following through with it is one of the challenges you will face. Coming up with funding and finding a competent team to help you realize this dream is only the beginning. However, knowing what you and your partners are willing to give to the practice plays a big part in the business venture's success. It is to your advantage to align yourself with the right people willing to "fight the good fight," understanding that there will be drawbacks and that, in the beginning, this new business you have created will dominate your life. The mindset and mental toughness required to reach the proverbial 'top' will help overcome the fear of risk and uncertainty. Your success depends on it!

These pages are structured to be easy-to-read, step-by-step processes you must follow in a specific order to better understand how to ensure your practice functions to its highest potential.

A brief overview of the chapters to follow:

Chapter 1: "Choosing The Right Staff" offers the team needed to ensure the business runs with minimal issues whether you are there or not. Frequently, business owners only remain as business owners rather than leaders because they want to know they are the reason the business functions. They relish that things fall apart when they are not around. Hoping that things fall apart without you is not the mindset of a person who wants their business to thrive. If you seek eventual financial freedom, the key is to teach the staff to care about the establishment as much as you do. Giving them the tools required involves reviewing resumes, credentials, and references BEFORE they walk through your doors.

Chapter 2, "Choosing The Right Practice Management Software," provides a detailed explanation of using the appropriate management system for your practice to comply with local and nationwide authorities and, of course, be as user-friendly as possible for your staff. It discusses that the software selected will be pricy. However, if chosen wisely, your return should supersede the cost.

Chapter 3: "Choosing The Right Script," gives a sample of what specific conversations should look like when your staff encounters a challenging confrontation with your patients. Their words and their delivery will determine the outcome of the end of the conversation. Make your staff understand that their being "right" or "wrong" is irrelevant during a patient dispute or encounter. The goal is to be direct but understand the patients' needs so that they want to return. They have many options; you need to be the obvious choice!

Chapter 4: "Policies & Procedures" is the less attractive topic. Still, knowing about them in detail is necessary to protect your investment. This chapter also includes key information and the importance of full transparency in your practice's financial policies. It is uncomfortable for most doctors to get involved in presenting this information, so it should be part of the intake process. The medical professional should not have to get involved with policy enforcement if they have selected the appropriate staff to carry out the task.

Chapter 5, "Know Your Technology & Resource Availability," highlights the government resources available to the public, especially physicians. They offer a plethora of research that many practices use as references. In addition, this chapter explores the rising popularity of AI-integrated technology that you should consider utilizing in your practice.

Chapter 6: "Have A Representative In All Departments." This chapter explains the importance of having a contact person who is a specialist in each section of your practice. This way, you are not depending solely on one individual; instead, you create individual accountability in the organization.

Chapter 7: "Decide Which Procedures To Do In-House Or At A Facility." This explores the numerous variables involved when deciding which procedures to perform within your practice or at an outside facility. One of the significant factors is cost. If the equipment needed to perform the service is not in demand or does not "pay you back," this is one of the details to consider before making a decision.

Chapter 8, "Run Reports," discusses another function of communicating your progress with your team. Suppose all your hard work does not show up in high numbers when you run a financial analysis. In that case, it is time to reconsider performing the service unless you choose to pick it as your "pro bono" service for the month or quarter.

Chapter 9: "Create surveys regularly." Surveys are what companies do now to engage. They allow the organization to know how the public perceives them. Knowing how to use that information will take some trial and error. However, the idea is to improve your practice through listening and learning.

Chapter 10: "Have Monthly Meetings." It is vital to communicate with your team and staff regularly. Monthly meetings are a great way to energize the team and discuss new or existing goals.

CHAPTER 1:

Choosing The

Right Staff

You opened a medical practice...now what?

The first thing to consider is who will lead the ship when you are away. Most business owners are genuinely concerned about what happens when they are away. It is your responsibility to select the right team who cares as much as you do about the life of the practice. The following leaders are essential for a medical practice to function:

<u>Your back office</u>
1) LPN/RN/MA
2) Nurse manager
3) Designated MD

For obvious reasons, the back-office staff is critical. They are the ones caring for your patients before they see you. How they behave and interact with the patients will determine the lifeline of your practice. Patients needing a more pleasant experience entering your doors will likely not return. In addition, they would be sure to leave a bad review via social media.

Depending on your practice type and size, having Medical Assistants, Licensed Practical Nurses, or Registered Nurses is essential. Here are the immediate differences between the three:

1. <u>**Licensed Practical Nurse (LPN)**</u>—Can perform primary nursing care to patients such as:
   - Monitoring vital signs
   - Breathing treatments
   - Hearing/vision tests
   - Phlebotomy
   - Patient health recording
   - Wound dressing
   - Catheter insertion

2. <u>**Registered Nurse (RN)**</u>—Can perform more complex care to patients, such as:
   - Administering medication
   - Administering vaccines
   - IV insertion
   - Creating or contributing to patient care plans

3. <u>**Medical Assistant (MA)**</u>—Can perform administrative and clinical duties (under supervision)
   - Prepare patients for examinations
   - Taking medical histories
   - Explaining treatment procedures to patients
   - Performing basic laboratory and in-office tests
   - Phlebotomy
   - Wound care and dressings

When choosing one of the above staff, the business owner must consider the practice's needs. The selection must benefit the business financially and functionally. They must be teachable, thorough, and capable of quickly following protocols and directions.

Nurse Manager

Having a nurse manager for your back office is a necessity. Their primary role is to support the nursing staff and instill protocols to prevent patient harm or negligence. In their executive position, they also serve as liaisons between the team and physicians when the challenge of embracing changes arises. Other responsibilities of your nurse manager include:

- Scheduling responsibilities
- Informing the physicians of statewide changes
- Keeping up with safety and compliance
- Ensuring that medical equipment maintenance is to company standards
- Confirming the presence of vaccine safety documentation

Designated MD

A designated medical doctor must be present on the premises. Contrary to popular belief, although employing a nurse practitioner has advantages, they require supervision under a medical doctor for all their scope of practice. Practices that do not adhere to these restrictions risk a hefty fine from the state.

Employing medical doctors with various specialties can be expensive but will pay off. Knowing the demographics of your practice's community will help you choose which specialty is necessary within your practice. For example, suppose your office is in a community with a significant prevalence of asthma. In that case, consider equipping your practice with an asthma specialist or an M.D. interested in the field. This detail of evaluating the needs of your community will guarantee a client base for your practice.

CHAPTER 2:

Choosing The Right Practice Management Software

<u>What is Practice Management?</u>

Practice Management (PM) enables medical practices and providers the capability of managing:

- Clinical charting
- Patient Intake
- Patient care
- Billing
- Revenue Cycle Management (RCM)
  Whatever PM software you choose must include customizable forms, e-prescribing capabilities, scheduling tools, real-time patient eligibility checks, and a patient portal. In addition, understanding the functionality of the programs provided within the software is pertinent to the successful implementation of proper use of the PM software. Below are details to look for when reviewing the installed programs in your software:

1. **<u>Clinical Charting</u>**-- is a complete record of a patient's clinical data and medical history. Such medical history should include the following:

- Demographics
- Vital signs

- Diagnoses
- Medications
- Allergies
- Lab/test results
- Treatment plans
- Immunization dates
- Progress notes

Systematic documentation of a patient's medical history relies on your ability to accurately chart your patient's treatment and overall care. It may be beneficial to remember that their records may be subject to insurance auditing or for legal purposes. Therefore, appropriate language must be a factor when charting medical history—even on phone notes!

2. **Patient Intake**—this is the process through which healthcare organizations use a platform to collect information before the patient's visit. Patient intake entails:

- Collection of demographics
- Collection of social and clinical data
- Production of consent forms
- Collection of insurance information
- Collection of payment

3. **Patient Care**-- refers to the prevention, evaluation, and management of common and uncommon illnesses while preserving the physical and mental well-being through services offered by healthcare professionals.

4. **Billing**-- is the process of accurately translating procedures performed by the provider to the appropriate codes to communicate with insurance providers.

5. **Revenue Cycle Management**---(RCM) Using medical billing software, healthcare facilities can improve patient care efficiency by tracking patient care episodes

from appointment scheduling to registration and account payment.

> The daily maintenance of a practice's revenue process should follow these nine steps:
> 1) Pre-registration
> 2) Registration
> 3) Charge capture
> 4) Utilization review
> 5) Coding
> 6) Claim submission
> 7) Remittance processing
> 8) Insurance follow-up
> 9) Patient collections.

<u>Pre-Registration</u>

Pre-registration is the collection of patient information before the visit. This collection consists of the patients':

Name

Address

Phone number/email address

Date of birth

Insurance information (identification number, policyholder)

Depending on the circumstances, the provider may want to know the patient's health history.

The entire pre-registration process should be done online at the patients' leisure. This implementation into your front office's workflow saves your practice time and prepares the patient for the office visit. They can then address any issues before coming into the office, such as past-due balances, inactive insurance, or failed pre-authorization required for a visit.

Registration

The registration process should go smoothly if your patients complete the pre-registration sent to them the day before. Therefore, all that remains is for them to verify that all information is accurate. This information includes the office's financial policy and the benefits' acknowledgment and assignment.

Charge Capture

Doctors and other healthcare providers use charge capture to record patient services. The practice must perform charge capture through electronic health systems. Electronic health records, or EHRs, are real-time, patient-centered records that make information available instantly and securely to authorized users (CMS.gov). Once the physician signs off on the chart, it is transmitted, reviewed, and processed for billing.

Coding

Healthcare facilities should all have an external scrubbing system. After the physician enters the procedures performed, they add the diagnoses and sign off on the chart for billing. However, before the claim gets sent to the insurance company, the biller must ensure that the Evaluation and Management codes they utilize contain no expired diagnoses. Taking the time to review this will ensure timely claims processing and payment.

Remittance Processing and Insurance Follow-Up

The health care payment and remittance advice transaction is the transmission of either:

1) Payment, with information about the transfer of funds and payment processing from a health plan to a health care provider's financial institution

OR

2) Explanation of benefits or remittance advice from a health plan to a health care provider (CMS.gov)

Remittance processing is vital to RCM's functionality. For instance, if the facility and insurance company agree that endoscopies will be reimbursed at $2000 in-network, but the remittance states otherwise, the biller should immediately escalate this to the insurance company's representative. The biller must take the same action if procedures are unpaid or payment is pending after a certain period.

Patient Collections

The front office must receive the patient's co-pay during service. Suppose they have a deductible AND a co-pay. In that case, the front office may deduct the co-pay from the estimated amount for the office visit. A standard amount should be expected and made available to the front desk for reference. In addition, there should always be a financial responsibility waiver signed by the guarantor and collected upfront. This workflow avoids unnecessary time spent on phone calls and more time focusing on today's patients.

As revenue cycle management expands, medical practices and facilities must work as one unit. For goals to exceed expectations, the process must unify all departments. Data must be accurate and adequately communicated, ensuring staff members know their responsibility to adhere to revenue cycles. Therefore, practice managers must eliminate inconsistencies from everyday functions.

Chapter 3:

Choosing The

Right Script

Having the staff representing your establishment is as important as teaching them the appropriate language. Customer service has never been more critical in the market today. If patients are unhappy with their treatment outcomes or, more urgently, how they felt after leaving your office, the odds of their returning are slim. The chances you have to recover an unhappy patient are minimal. Therefore, every opportunity to coach your staff on the importance of delivery should be taken advantage of.

Creating a script for every possible scenario is one way to eliminate the risk of losing potential clients. Below is a list of issues you may encounter and the appropriate techniques:

1) A patient calls demanding to speak with a doctor who is not in the office. Your staff explained that they were out of the office, but other doctors were available. They are still not happy; no other doctor will understand their case.

Response: "I understand your frustration (Last name of patient), but our medical records are systematically designed for these situations. The notes are highly detailed, and our doctors constantly review their prior visits to ensure they know about their patients' conditions. May I have Dr._____ reach out to you?"

This approach is usually practical. The patient feels assured that all the doctors are on board with their treatment plan and needs. That is ultimately the patient's primary concern; they want to avoid going over their medical history with another doctor every time they call your office.

2) "I have a high deductible. How do I know what I'll be charged every time I come in for a sick visit?"

   Response: "Unfortunately, every visit is unique and billed based on multiple factors. When lab tests are performed in or out of the office, the severity of the visit can affect the deductible amount applied by your insurance company."
   Explaining that the insurance company sets the rates takes the ownership away from your practice. Remind your staff that most patients need help understanding insurance terminology. Keep it as simple as possible, and ensure your tone is welcoming and not condescending.

3) "My other office never charged me for missing appointments! All you people want is money!"

   Response: "I am so sorry it seems that way; this is not our intention. We are a popular practice; when a patient misses their appointment, it inconveniences other patients. We would not want you to wait unnecessarily, which is why our office has enforced this policy."

When you highlight that it's about the patients and not only you (while also highlighting that you are well-known and in high demand), they tend to understand better why your practice enforces this policy.

Revise your scripts as often as possible so that your staff and new staff members have a reference if they encounter these issues.

Chapter 4:

Policies &

Procedures

Every professional business needs to have policies and procedures set in place. These systems ensure consistency whether you, as the manager, are in the building. It would benefit your company to have these policies and procedures clearly written and easily accessible to the staff. Examples of what your "policy bible" should contain are as follows:

1) Waivers
2) Financial Policies
3) HIPAA guidelines
4) No-show Policies
5) Office Policies

Waivers

Why do we need waivers?

The primary purpose of waivers is to protect your practice and the patients. It helps them decide whether they would like specific procedures to be performed by you, the risks, and their financial responsibilities. Before and after the procedure/testing, they should know what to expect, and your practice should get reimbursed for the services performed. Every practice has waivers tailored to their needs. However, there are essential items that must be presented as a disclaimer to your patients:

1) An informative statement of the services you are providing
2) The self-pay rate if insurance does not cover
3) The patient's name, date of birth, and date of procedure
4) The procedure code with a description
5) The patient's consent with signature

Financial Policies

Similarly to waivers, a copy of your financial policy must be readily available for patients to see at every visit. These policies should highlight the following:

1) Credit card use
2) Co-pays and deductibles
3) Referrals and pre-authorization
4) Missed appointments
5) Self-pay patients
6) Medical records fees
7) Outstanding balances and payment plan options
8) Special fees billed to insurance companies and patient responsibilities

HIPAA guidelines

What is HIPAA?
"The Health Insurance Portability and Accountability Act of 1996 (HIPAA) is a federal law requiring national standards to protect sensitive patient health information from being disclosed without the patient's consent or knowledge. The U.S. Department of Health and Human Services (HHS) issued the HIPAA Privacy Rule to

implement the requirements of HIPAA. The HIPAA Security Rule protects a subset of information covered by the Privacy Rule." (CDC)

You are responsible for ensuring that the official definition of HIPAA and the patient's check-in routine are posted clearly in the office. The HIPAA requirement should also include who the patient will give access to for their medical records and to whom they will disclose test results.

No-Show Policies

As is standard procedure in medical offices, patients who do not cancel an appointment with at least 24 hours' notice or do not attend the visit are considered no-shows. Estimated no-show rates are 5-7%. While this may seem low, it decreases revenue, costs, and staff time and can affect patient results.

Following are some tips that may provide some guidance on billing management for patient no-shows:

- Always review patient contracts before billing no-show charges. For instance, Medicare patients can be billed directly, but providers will not receive Medicare payments. In addition, all patients (regardless of insurance coverage) should be priced the same, prohibiting Medicare patients from discrimination.
- Post your no-show fee policy on your website, in your office, and on patient paperwork, such as appointment reminders. Also, staff should verbally communicate the no-show policy to patients.
- Create a workflow where your staff is alerted to follow up with patients who have missed appointments. They should advise patients why keeping appointments is vital for consistency in treatment. Of course, there should be exceptions for emergencies.

- Document no-shows and follow-up calls in the patient's file. Communication is key.
- Ensure scheduling systems can record no-shows. Medical providers typically schedule 15-minute appointments, while new patient visits could take 30-45 minutes. When no-show rates or slow periods appear, book two 15-minute segments, allowing the remaining 30 minutes for longer appointments or new patients.
- Suppose a patient is billed a no-show fee on a credit card; your billing management system should assess this self-pay charge using a miscellaneous dummy code.

The type of patients a practice has can also affect the no-show percentage. Specialists whose services are not covered by insurance or Medicaid are vulnerable to no-shows. Some practices charge a no-show fee when feasible, but that has its challenges. Medicaid does not allow a provider to bill a patient for missed appointments. Whatever method you use to advise patients of the consequences of no-shows, make it clear and concise and communicate effectively. Train your staff accordingly on their duties in dealing with no-shows. Properly communicating expectations with the staff will assist in creating a thriving, beneficial practice for you and your patients.

Chapter 5: Know Your Technology & Resource Availability

With the aging population and exposure to new diseases, having up-to-date equipment in your office/facility is crucial. In addition, moving away from the usage of standard machinery will speed up the visits and ensure accuracy. Some examples of technology to consider introducing into your practice include:

1. Electronic Vital Signs Devices
- Must have the ability to check blood pressure, heart rate, and temperature

2. Portable Vision and Hearing Devices
- Must support state guidelines
- Must require minimal training to use
- Driverless printing capabilities
- Clear and efficient results

3. Stationary and portable computers/iPads

4. Shared Devices—these allow multiple users to access data at the same time:
- Cloud storage
- Database server

The advantage of having up-to-date types of equipment in your office or facility is limitless. It allows physicians to respond rapidly to identify patient needs, provide prompt intervention, and improve modes of communication. Also, medication error prevention is achieved by providing physicians with point-of-care decision support with accessible references.

The companies that many facilities purchase these devices from vary by popularity and cost. It is essential to do your research before buying from these companies. Some companies offer demonstrations of how their platforms would integrate with your current devices, and professionals are presented with the option of several types of services the platforms provide. Below are a few government websites that discuss new technology as well as resources for research:

1. National Institutes of Health (NIH)
2. Agency For Healthcare Research And Quality (AHRQ)
3. Centers For Medicare And Medicaid Services (CMS)

National Institutes of Health- According to its missions and goals, the NIH is one of the world's foremost medical research centers today. An agency of the Department of Health and Human Services, the NIH is the Federal focal point for health research. (NIH)
The goals of the agency are:

- To foster fundamental creative discoveries, innovative research strategies, and their applications as a basis to advance significantly the Nation's capacity to protect and improve health;

- To develop, maintain, and renew scientific human and physical resources that will assure the Nation's capability to prevent disease;

- To expand the knowledge base in medical and associated sciences to enhance the Nation's economic well-being and ensure a continued high return on the public investment in research and

- To exemplify and promote the highest level of scientific integrity, public accountability, and social responsibility in the conduct of science. (NIH)

Being that the NIH is government-funded, this can benefit your practice by being ahead of medical research and technological advancement as it pertains to your practice.

<u>Agency For Healthcare Research And Quality</u>-The Agency for Healthcare Research and Quality's (AHRQ) mission is to produce evidence to make health care safer, higher quality, more accessible, equitable, and affordable, and to work within the U.S. Department of Health and Human Services and with other partners to make sure that the evidence is understood and used. (Quality) The main goals of AHRQ:

- Invest in research on the Nation's health delivery system, such as:

a) Project ECHO (Extension for Community Healthcare Outcomes), which trains and supports primary care clinicians in rural communities to provide specialized care for their patients. This model has flourished, receiving ongoing funding from the State of New Mexico, spreading to other States, and expanding from its initial focus on hepatitis C into new clinical areas, including mental health and substance abuse and HIV. The Veterans Health Administration has also adopted it to expand veterans' access to high-quality care nationwide. (Quality)

b) AHRQ's Re-Engineered Discharge (RED) is a structured protocol and suite of implementation tools that help hospitals rework their discharge processes to reduce readmissions by determining patients' needs and carefully designing and communicating discharge plans. Hospitals using these tools have seen a 30 percent reduction in hospital readmissions and emergency room visits. (Quality)

- Create materials to teach and train healthcare systems and professionals to put the research results into practice:

a) AHRQ supported the development of the Comprehensive Unit-based Safety Program (CUSP), a highly effective method of preventing healthcare-associated infections (HAIs). CUSP combines improved safety culture, teamwork, and communication with a checklist of proven practices for preventing HAIs. AHRQ has promoted the use of CUSP in a series of nationwide projects that addressed various HAIs and produced CUSP toolkits to help clinicians prevent these infections. CUSP was implemented in over 1,000 U.S. intensive care units (ICUs) to prevent deadly central line-associated bloodstream infections (CLABSI). ICUs that used CUSP methods and tools were able to reduce these bloodstream infections by 41 percent, preventing over 2,100 CLABSI cases, saving more than 500 lives, and avoiding more than $36 million in excess costs. CUSP tools are free and available on the AHRQ website, and they can be adapted and used based on the specific setting. (Quality)

b) In 2015, AHRQ launched an initiative to directly bring the latest scientific research, tools, and support to over 5,000 primary care physicians to improve the care of over 8 million Americans. AHRQ awarded seven large grants to establish EvidenceNOW, an initiative aligned with Million Hearts® that will provide practice support to over 5,000 primary care physicians to improve the heart health of millions of patients and improve the capacity of the practices to incorporate new research findings and information into practice. (Quality)

- Generate measures and data used by providers and policymakers:

a) AHRQ created and maintained the gold-standard suite of surveys called the Consumer Assessment of Healthcare Providers and Systems, which validly assesses patients' care experience in hospitals, nursing homes, and doctors' offices. The hospital industry, patients, and CMS chose the hospital version of the AHRQ survey to measure all patient experience elements for CMS' Hospital Quality Initiative. CMS incorporates these results into the Hospital Compare Web tool and its five-star rating system. (Quality)

AHRQ's <u>Medical Expenditure Panel Survey</u> data helped the Medicaid and CHIP Payment and Access Commission develop estimates of eligibility for Medicaid and the Children's Health Insurance Program; the Congressional Budget Office also uses AHRQ data in its estimates of the budgetary impact of many Congressional proposals. (Quality)

Centers For Medicare and Medicaid Services- CMS is the federal agency that provides over 160 million health coverage through Medicare, Medicaid, the Children's Health Insurance Program, and the Health Insurance Marketplace. CMS works in partnership with the entire healthcare community to improve quality, equity, and outcomes in the healthcare system. (CMS)

CMS is the beast of government programs. Their functions include a wide range such as:

- Compliance and enforcement of health insurance market reforms:

a) Title XXVII of the Public Health Service Act (PHS Act) contemplates that states will exercise primary enforcement authority over health insurance issuers in the group and individual markets to ensure compliance with health insurance market reforms. If a state notifies the Centers for Medicare & Medicaid Services that it does not have statutory authority to enforce or that it is not otherwise enforcing one or more of the provisions of title XXVII, or if CMS determines that the state is not substantially enforcing the requirements, CMS has the responsibility to implement these provisions in the state. This enforcement framework, which has been in place since 1996, ensures that consumers in all states have protections under the Affordable Care Act and other parts of the PHS Act. (CMS)

b) States and CMS have worked closely to ensure compliance with the federal law's health insurance accountability and consumer protections. The vast majority of states are enforcing the Affordable Care Act health insurance market reforms. Some states lack the authority, the ability to implement these provisions, or both. CMS is responsible for enforcing these requirements in a state that is not enforcing the health insurance market reforms either through a collaborative arrangement with the state or by direct enforcement to ensure all residents of the state receive the protections of the Affordable Care Act. (CMS)

c) Collect and analyze data, produce research reports, and work to eliminate fraud and abuse within the healthcare system. (Investopedia)

d) To provide a healthcare system with better care, access to coverage, and improved health. (Investopedia)

e) Releases updated Medicare premium and deductible information each year. (Investopedia)

Knowing the functionalities of each of these programs is essential. They provide valuable data for specific practice implementations, policy enforcement, and updated downloadable forms in your office or facility.

<u>Artificial Intelligence In Your Practice</u>

Artificial intelligence has become widely used because of its time-reducing advantages. Nothing is more valuable than time for a specialist or surgeon in the medical field. Integrating AI-powered devices like stethoscopes is used more frequently in private practices and facilities today. Unlike traditional stethoscopes, the AI-powered stethoscope may be used in noisy environments, and the readings can be obtained by anyone with permitted access to the patient's medical records. Other notable applications for AI in your practice are listed below :

a) <u>Medical Records review</u>- the purpose of this service is to justify procedures to insurance companies to obtain authorization or determine the best course of action in treating patients with complicated cases.

How AI can help

Using algorithms, AI can read, categorize, and index the data inputted by experts. As with all things, the tools are as good as the user. If the information inputted is inaccurate or faulty, so will the outcome of the data.

b) <u>Medical Coding-</u> associates alpha-numerical characters with procedures, diagnoses, and medical equipment based on the physician's documentation. The services must be performed in a registered professional environment to be eligible for billing.

How AI can help

AI can easily decipher the documentation, extract keywords while analyzing patterns, and translate this into medical codes for billing in minutes.

c) <u>Chart Documentation</u>—Chart documentation details the specifics of clinical care provided to patients. These records allow other clinicians to learn the patient's history and give each individual the best possible treatment.

How AI can help

The physician can use speech-to-text, and the AI-powered technology can act as a "scribe" and transform into comprehensive chart notes for the patient's medical records, making it easy to interpret if other physicians and providers view the chart or take over the patient's care.

It is no secret that technology is fast-moving and integrating into the medical world. As advanced technology has many advantages, it is crucial to recognize that a machine cannot replace basic human needs. It would be best to determine how to leverage these advantages while still maintaining a warm, patient atmosphere and a place where employees want to work.

Chapter 6: Have A Representative In All Departments

As you grow your practice, you will find the value of having a contact in each department. Having a representative for specific departments acts as a liaison, protects your business, and aids in appointing accountability to a responsible individual, hopefully resulting in minimal errors or unnecessary fines. Examples of types of representatives required are as follows:

1) *Patient representative*
2) *Insurance representative*
3) *In-Office Compliance Officer*

Patient Representatives- the purpose of having a representative is to provide warmth, support, and attention to your patients before and after their office visit. Their primary function is addressing patients' issues, such as insurance difficulties, gathering medical records and information pertinent to their care, or simply providing psychological or emotional support. In addition, they should meet the following qualifications before being appointed to this role:

1) Have extensive knowledge of medical terminology and insurance benefits

2) Knowledge of the specialty that you provide so that they can intelligently advise patients if they have follow-up questions

3) The ability to multitask and the skill to complete tasks promptly

4) Strong interpersonal and communicative skills

5) Appointment coordination

6) Provide counsel on treatment options available to patients

Insurance Representatives- are employed by insurance companies and are known as "Provider Service Representatives." Their main goal is to assist medical providers in understanding their relationships (and contracts) with specific insurance companies.
They present as advocates to the providers, but it should be remembered that, ultimately, they do not work for you. Although these representatives are employees of the insurance companies, it is advantageous to build a rapport with them as they know precisely how to get you in touch with specific departments when handling authorizations for medical equipment, prescriptions, or procedures. Some reps may even know who to speak with to waive certain charges for your patients in a dispute.

In-Office Compliance Officers- are responsible for ensuring everyone in your office fully complies with the rules and regulations established by your local and state agencies. They perform as a proactive measure to help avoid the company getting fined, and they help develop ethics and a code of conduct. How they function in your business include but are not limited to the following:

1) Ensuring that all patient records have signed and dated HIPPA forms

2) Ensuring that there are waivers for every procedure, especially if they are usually an uncovered service by most insurance companies

3) Ensuring that the language in each medical record is legally appropriate, easy to read, and accessible upon request by patients or insurance companies

4) Ensure that physicians' and specific personnel's licenses, certifications, and permits are valid and up-to-date.

5) Hold monthly meetings on compliance adherence and risk management with all staff members

6) Offer training and educational requirements to current and new employees

7) Conduct monthly internal monitoring and auditing.

Who can you appoint as your compliance officer?

It is recommended that a board member in your company be assigned this role. This could be a senior physician, a CFO, or, if you choose, a general counsel. Whoever you choose should communicate directly with the CEO and Board of Directors, have high integrity, and be able to foster the company culture.

Chapter 7: Decide Which Procedures To Do In-house Or At A Facility

Many variables must be considered when determining whether to perform specific procedures in your office or direct the patient to an outside facility. One of the obvious variables is the cost to perform the procedure in-house. If the equipment cost does not "pay you back" per se, it would benefit you and the practice to refer the patient elsewhere. Here are some factors to review before making a final decision:

1) What is your specialty? Is the procedure typically performed by physicians practicing your specialty, or can the patient go anywhere?
   a) What sets you apart from other facilities?
   b) Are the wait times for the test results in your practice the same as if the patient went to another facility?
   c) Are your fees higher or lower than others?

2) Do you own the equipment? Or is this a rental that you would have to pay each month?

3) If insurance does not typically cover this test, what resources do you make available to the patient?

4) Does your biller know the correct procedure and diagnosis code needed to bill the service?

5) Do you have the documents required in the patient's medical record that justifies medical necessity?

   a) If not, do you know the steps to take to get them?

6) How often will the equipment maintenance need to be performed?

   a) What are the costs associated with the maintenance?

Some standard services should always be available to your patients. The procedures you provide, such as specified blood tests, radiological procedures, etc., are convenient when done in-house. You will find that the idea of a "one-stop shop" for existing and potential patients in your establishment is an invaluable solution to multiple dilemmas you may face.

Chapter 8: Run Reports

Running biweekly reports should become part of your practice's routine. The benefits of enforcing this habit will be exponentially apparent when determining what services are being appropriately reimbursed by the most common insurance companies and self-pay patients. For example, suppose insurance companies refuse to pay for a particular service. How would you and your team be made aware? It would not be presented to you and your team without report generation.

In addition, upon signing your contract with the insurance companies, there are basic procedures they agree to pay at a certain percentage. Without running weekly, biweekly, or monthly reports, it would not be known whether they are holding up their end of the deal. Running reports will also give you an idea of whether sending patients to outside facilities would be beneficial instead of performing the procedures in your practice. The self-pay options should be reviewed if the procedure is standard or pertinent to your specialty.

No Fancy Required!

Contrary to popular belief, no "fancy," overpriced programs are required to run these biweekly reports. One of the minimal functions of the Practice Management (PM) software you choose should be able to run reports quickly (without contacting IT for support). Things you should input and filter to run an efficient analysis are as follows:

1) The correct Current Procedural Terminology (CPT®) codes and International Diseases of Classification (ICD-10) codes

   a) Can be multiple procedure/diagnosis codes and add-on codes

2) Insurance companies you have billed to

3) Appropriate codes for place of service

4) A realistic date range for proper analysis

A knowledgeable billing team must ensure these reports are run and analyzed regularly. Remember that the reports will not help you if nothing is done with the information.

As with all things, an action plan must be set into place if processes are not producing the results you desire. Examples of what an action plan should look like:

1) A simple spreadsheet with columns to indicate insurance company payments versus denials with procedure codes and diagnoses

   a) Denial reasons
   b) Group by insurance company

Once this information is gathered, your team can create another spreadsheet or a simple list indicating the steps necessary to get paid for the services or ways to transition from doing the procedure in-house. The action plan aims to come to a resolution and provide a clear roadmap for you and your team to provide the best service to your patients without compromising your value.

No rule states you can't care for your patients and be adequately compensated at the same time!

Chapter 9: Create surveys regularly

Although some people find surveys annoying, they can be effective in your practice. Most companies limit surveys to just the clients they serve, but you will create a system where surveys are generated to be used internally within your organization. This will ensure satisfaction amongst your employees and your current or potential patients.

Why use surveys?

1) **They allow anonymity.** Anonymity gives people a sense of safety when they can say how they feel without fearing judgment or argument.

2) **They create exposure.** When starting a new business, exposure is the key to being found. Since surveys can be accessed by virtually anyone, anywhere, at any time, you can reach new audiences with few limitations.

3) **Make data analysis easy.** Using the right program that fits your needs, you will obtain scalable results for proper analyses, which will diagnose any shortcomings your practice may have.

4) **They allow you to target a specific audience.**

Your targeted audience should serve a purpose for your research. Creating random questions that give you no answers to the questions you seek would be a waste of your time and the audience. For instance, if you aim to learn new or better ways to make your scheduling process more user-friendly, tailoring specific questions to the audience would be the way to achieve this goal. Sometimes, a simple question such as,' How was your visit today?' could put your business on the map, especially if their response is positive.

Automating these administrative tasks will be vital to your practice's daily functioning. It is easy to fall into the safety net of "easy" by simply asking your patients to leave a positive review. But, in the grand scheme, you are looking for a lucrative business with longevity. You must be willing to hear the bad with the good to improve on all levels to achieve this goal.

Chapter 10: Have monthly meetings

Engagement with your staff and colleagues should always be your number one priority. They help you function as a whole. So, knowing your staff and showing that you care through listening to suggestions will catapult your business.

As stated earlier, the key to a fruitful, pleasant environment is having people around you who care as much as you do about the business's success. Monthly meetings will allow you to perform a temperature check on where your team is with the company goals. They are also an opportunity to energize the team to discuss implementations, raises, or staff recognition.

Whether mandating staff reviews or having a conversation, this alignment can be achieved as long as it remains consistent. You must prioritize and devote at least thirty minutes of listening! If, at the end of your meetings, everyone is synonymous with upholding the company standards and maintaining integrity while keeping the culture alive and your

patients happy, you have hit your target!

Make this a fun, engaging, themed event, not a dreaded one. Think of a fun game to play with the staff that makes them feel included while making it a learning experience.

Chapter 11: Conclusion

Starting a medical practice is a courageous move. Congratulations on your strength in following these guidelines to make it a reality!

There are many medical practices available to the public. But knowing why you started your practice and how to remain relevant while being compliant will give you an advantage over your competitors.

Starting a medical practice will be a rigorous and lonely path. There will be some months, in the beginning, where you will question every decision you have made and regret it. But remember the 'cliché' that nothing is easy and success is a gift you earn with consistency. Don't try to reinvent the wheel! Especially when just beginning, you will be wise to do the things that are a proven success.

Only take those along with you who share the same vision and are ready and willing to sacrifice, lose sleep, and spend money on the fully actualized dream! You got this!

References

CDC. (2022, June 27). *Centers for Disease Control and Prevention*. Retrieved April 7, 2023

CMS, C. F. (2023, September). *https://www.cms.gov/about-cms*. Retrieved February 24, 2024

Investopedia. (n.d.).
https://www.investopedia.com/terms/u/us-centers-medicare-and-medicaid-services-cms.asp. Retrieved February 27, 2024

NIH. (2015, July 7). *nih.gov*. Retrieved November 17, 2023

Quality, A. F. (2022, July).
https://www.ahrq.gov/cpi/about/profile/index.html. Retrieved February 24, 2024

About the Author

With over 20 years of experience in the medical field, Dee Whitelocke has made a name for herself in the Medical Billing and Coding industry. Dee Whitelocke has consulted and helped hundreds of practices after deciding to become a company owner just three years ago. Whitelocke gives back to the community by offering virtual mini-tutorial classes on the basics of billing and coding free of charge. An advocate of mindset, she monitors a Facebook group with her team: Mindset Over Matter...with no selling or pitches involved, just a group of like-minded individuals with uplifting quotes, videos, and stories to share.

Stay tuned for more of Dee Whitelocke's work!